Nursing & Health Survival Guide

Cancer Care

Ian Peate

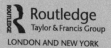

T0033790

Routledge
Taylor & Francis Group

LONDON AND NEW YORK

First published 2012 by Pearson Education Limited

Published 2014 by Routledge
2 Park Square, Milton Park, Abingdon, Oxon OX14 4RN
7 11 Third Avenue, New York, NY 10017, USA

Routledge is an imprint of the Taylor & Francis Group, an informa business

Copyright © 2012, Taylor & Francis.

The right of Ian Peate to be identified as author of this Work has been asserted
by him in accordance with the Copyright, Designs and Patents Act 1988.

All rights reserved. No part of this book may be reprinted or reproduced or utilised in any
by any electronic, mechanical, or other means, now known or hereafter invented, includir
photocopying and recording, or in any information storage or retrieval system, without pe
in writing from the publishers.

Notices
Knowledge and best practice in this field are constantly changing. As new research and
broaden our understanding, changes in research methods, professional practices, or me
treatment may become necessary.

Practitioners and researchers must always rely on their own experience and knowledge in
evaluating and using any information, methods, compounds, or experiments described h
using such information or methods they should be mindful of their own safety and the saf
others, including parties for whom they have a professional responsibility.

To the fullest extent of the law, neither the Publisher nor the authors, contributors, or edit
assume any liability for any injury and/or damage to persons or property as a matter of pr
liability, negligence or otherwise, or from any use or operation of any methods, products,
instructions, or ideas contained in the material herein.

ISBN : 978-1-4479-1204-0 (hbk)

British Library Cataloguing-in-Publication Data
A catalogue record for this book is available from the British Library

Library of Congress Cataloging-in-Publication Data
Peate, Ian.
    Cancer care / Ian Peate.
        p. ; cm. -- (Nursing & health survival guide)
    Includes bibliographical references.
    ISBN 978-1-4479-1204-0 (pbk.)
    I. Title. II. Series: Nursing & health survival guides.
    [DNLM: 1. Neoplasms--nursing--Handbooks. WY 49]

616.99'40231--dc23

                                                    2012006036

Typeset in 8/9.5pt Helvetica by 35

contents

While effort has been made to ensure that the content of this guide is accurate, no responsibility will be taken for inaccuracies, omissions or errors. This is a guide only. The information is provided solely on the basis that readers will be responsible for making their own assessment and adhering to organisation policy of the matters discussed therein. The author does not accept liability to any person for the information obtained from this publication or loss or damages incurred as a result of reliance upon the material contained in this guide.

publisher's acknowledgements

We are grateful to the following for permission to reproduce copyright material:

Figures

Figures on pages 6 and 17 from Colbert, Bruce J.; Ankey, Jeff J.; Lee, Karen, *Anatomy and Physiology for Health Professionals: An Interactive Journey*, 1st © 2007, Printed and Electronically reproduced by permission of Pearson Education, Inc., Upper Saddle River, New Jersey; Figure on page 7 from http://www.macmillan.org.uk/Cancerinformation/Aboutcancer/Whatiscancer.aspx, Crush/agencyrush.com; Figure on page 8 from illustration by Cell Imaging Core of the Center for Reproductive Sciences © Copyright reserved: University of Kansas, USA, www.kumc.edu; Figure on page 13 from diagram © EMIS 2012 as distributed at http://www.patient.co.uk/health/Cancer-What-are-Cancer-and-Tumours?.htm; Figure on page 21 from Copyright © Cancer Research UK. Taken from http://info.cancerresearchuk.org

In some instances we have been unable to trace the owners of copyright material, and we would appreciate any information that would enable us to do so.

Understanding cancer is essential if you are to help the patients you care for. Every two minutes somebody is diagnosed with cancer. Cancer is one the biggest killers in the UK. Over 250,000 people are diagnosed with cancer killing over 130,000 per year, remaining one of the central priorities for the NHS. The most common cancers in the UK are:

- lung
- prostate
- breast
- bowel (also known as colorectal cancer)

Cancer is the biggest killer worldwide and deaths associated with cancer are predicted to rise. Even if we do not develop cancer ourselves we are sure to know relatives or friends who have cancer. Cancer affects all of us.

Cancer is becoming more understood with more people being treated successfully but, cancer remains one of the most feared diseases. The term cancer can bring about feelings of hopelessness and helplessness in patients and sometimes in the people who care for them.

Cancer can be disruptive and in many cases it is a life-threatening process that can have an impact on the whole person as well as that individual's family and their friends. The role and function of the nurse must be based on the understanding that cancer is a chronic condition that has acute occurrences. Often the patient is treated as an outpatient and is typically treated with a combination of therapies.

Just as important, the nurse must acknowledge that when caring for the person with cancer this involves:

- health education
- early detection
- treatment
- supportive care

There will be long-term follow-up and in a number of instances end of life care.

Defining cancer

The term cancer is used for diseases in which abnormal cells divide without control, and can invade other tissues; in essence, a disruption in the regulation of growth of healthy cells occurs. Cells proliferate without normal organisation or normal control; cellular function becomes distorted, this is called carcinogenesis.

Cancer cells spread to other parts of the body through blood and lymph systems: this is known as metastases. The abnormal cells (the mutations) migrate from their original site invading nearby tissues and forming masses at distant sites of the body. Much progress related to unravelling the various steps associated with the processes related to carcinogenesis has occurred.

Cancer is a general term describing a group of related diseases. Every case of cancer is unique, with its own group of genetic changes and growth properties: it is essential to remember that the people who have cancer and their families are also unique. There are many main types of cancer. Cancer can be grouped into broader categories.

GROUP	FORMATION	EXAMPLE
Carcinoma	Cancer beginning in the skin or tissues that line or cover internal organs	• Lung • Colon
Sarcoma	Cancer beginning in the bone, cartilage, fat, muscle, blood vessels or other connective or supportive tissue; these are rare	• Kaposi's sarcoma • Fibrosarcoma

GROUP	FORMATION	EXAMPLE
Leukaemia	Cancer starting in the blood forming tissues such as the bone marrow, causes large numbers of abnormal blood cells to be produced; they then enter the blood stream	• Acute lymphoblastic leukaemia • Chronic myeloid leukaemia
Lymphoma	Cancer beginning in the cells of the immune system	• Non-Hodgkin lymphoma
Central nervous system	Cancers beginning in the tissues of the brain and spinal cord	• Astrocytoma • Intramedullary tumour

There are a number of other terms used to describe cancer, for example, malignancy, tumour, neoplasm.

■ THE NATURE OF CANCER

Cancer is not a single disease: it is an umbrella term.

- There are hundreds of different types and sub types of cancer affecting young and older people.
- Almost every tissue or organ in the body has the capacity to develop the disease.
- There is no age group, ethnicity or gender resistant to cancer; these features play a role in the incidence of some particular cancers, frequency and severity.

Cancer can have an overwhelming emotional and physical impact on the individual and is associated with significant complications (morbidity) and potential death (mortality).

Some cancers grow quickly; others can take years to become a threat to the patient. There are differences between cases of cancer, even of those of same organ (for example, different cases of breast cancer); this is one of the main reasons why treatment can be so difficult.

In spite of the differences between various types of cancer, all cancers share some common characteristics. It is necessary to understand the basic, shared, features of cancer as this will allow for an understanding of detection, diagnosis and the possible treatment options.

■ THE BIOLOGY OF CANCER

The development of cancer is a complex process involving the disruption of the regulation of the growth of normal cells. In order to begin to understand cancer it is important to appreciate normal cell growth and regulation. We are all made up of approximately a hundred million million (100,000,000,000,000) cells; there are over 200 various types of cells in the body. The cells cluster together forming tissue; tissues make up organs such as the breast, lung, prostate and colon.

Cells are formed from chemicals and other structures and found in all living matter. Almost all cells are microscopic, varying in size, shape and purpose. Cells are the building blocks of the body providing proper functioning for processes required to sustain life, for example, digestion, respiration, reproduction. This is a typical cell and its components:

Cellular components

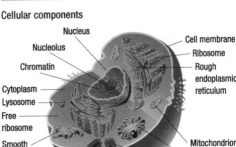

Source: from Colbert, B.J., Ankey, J. and Lee, K.T. *Anatomy and Physiology for Health Professionals. An Interactive Journey, 1st* © 2007. Printed and electronically reproduced by permission of Pearson Education, Inc., Upper Saddle River, New Jersey.

At any one time the majority of cells in the body are not dividing, but they become stimulated to enter a cycle of division by growth factors or hormones (chemical messengers produced by the body, influencing the growth of certain cancers); this eventually results in the cell dividing into two daughter cells. Cells within different tissues are highly specialised and have a role to play, doing a specific job.

- Control of the cell cycle occurs through chemicals which combine with and activate enzymes.
- Some chemical messengers trigger a 'braking' action stopping the cycle from proceeding.
- There are a number of points during the cell cycle ensuring it proceeds in the right order. If there are any deviations, apoptosis (cell death) occurs.

- If there is a malfunction of any regulators of cell growth a division can result causing a rapid proliferation of immature cells.

CANCER CELLS

Normal body cells have a number of important characteristics. They can:

- reproduce themselves precisely
- stop reproducing at the right time
- remain together in the right place
- self-destruct if they become damaged
- become specialised or 'mature'

Cells are said to be able to reproduce up to 50 or 60 times as a maximum, after this they die. Cancer cells are different: they do not die, they migrate to another part of the body, continuing to reproduce; for example, one cell becomes 2, then 4, and then 8, and then 16, and then 32 and so on:

- Cancer cells keep on doubling, irrespective of the damage the extra cells cause to the part of the body where the cancer is growing.

Cells forming tumour

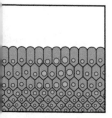 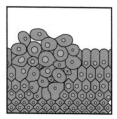

Normal cells   Cells forming a tumour

Source: Macmillan Cancer Support

- Normal cells cease maturation once they have been made
- Cancer cells do not specialise, but stay immature.

As a result of the rapid replication some of the genetic information in the cell can become lost and the cells become more and more unsophisticated with a tendency to reproduce faster and even more indiscriminately.

Differentiation

Cells usually become specialised during their development. All cells undergo an important adjustment during their lifetime, moving from unspecialised cells undergoing growth into specific cell types performing the responsibilities of specific tissues and organs: this is called differentiation – a less specialised cell becomes a more specialised cell. Cells originate from 'stem' cells; as the embryo grows, these cells differentiate, taking on different shapes in order to fulfil specific roles:

Cell differentiation

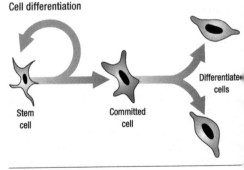

Stem cell

Committed cell

Differentiated cells

Source: The Center for Reproductive Sciences

Differentiation radically alters a cell's size, shape, membrane potential, metabolic activity and the cell's responsiveness to signals (usually hormonal signalling).

- If more than 75% of the tissue has altered this is poorly differentiated or undifferentiated; most of it has become altered and cancerous.
- If only 50% of the tissue has changed, this is moderately differentiated.
- If less than 25% has changed this is known as minimal differentiation.

This is important because it can help to determine how progressive the disease is; it also impacts on a person's cancer diagnosis. The more the tissue has changed, the less likely it is to respond positively to cancer treatment.

■ SECTION SUMMARY

There are a variety of types of cells in the body and there are different types of cancer, arising from different types of cells. Cancers can arise from any tissue. What is important to understand is that usually there are notable differences between different types of cancer:

- some cancers develop and spread faster than others
- some are easier to treat than others, especially if they are diagnosed at an early stage
- some respond better than other cancers to chemotherapy, radiotherapy, or other treatments
- for some people there is a very good possibility of being cured; however, for others the outlook is poor

So, cancer is not just one condition. When caring for people with cancer it is essential to understand:

- what type of cancer has developed
- the size
- if there is any spread
- how well the specific type of cancer responds to the various types of treatments

Understanding cancer biology can often be daunting. You should spend a little more time in developing your understanding of cell biology, then relate this to cancer cell biology; this will help you feel more confident when caring for people with cancer.

Tumours

A tumour can be described as a lump or growth of tissue made up from abnormal cells. Tumours are divided into two types, benign and malignant. Cancer is the name given to a malignant tumour.

■ BENIGN TUMOURS

These can form in many parts of the body, growing at a slow rate, not spreading to or invading other tissues. These tumours are:

- not cancerous
- not typically life-threatening

Left alone they do not usually cause any harm, but some benign tumours can cause problems. If the benign tumour grows and becomes large this can result in local pressure symptoms or the size can look unsightly. Some benign tumours arise in cells in hormone glands, for example, the thyroid gland causing excess production of hormones resulting in unwanted effects. What hormones are produced in the following glands?

GLAND	HORMONE(S) PRODUCED
Pituitary	
Thyroid	
Adrenal	
Ovaries	
Testes	
Pancreas	

MALIGNANT TUMOURS

Malignant tumours are called cancers and:
- tend to grow quickly
- enter neighbouring tissues and organs causing damage
- can spread beyond the original area, destroying tissues

A primary tumour refers to the original site where a tumour first develops.

Malignant tumours can spread and break away from the primary site to other parts of the body forming secondary tumours, known as metastatic spread (metastases).

Secondary malignant tumours can grow, break away and damage tissues close by and spread again through the bloodstream or lymphatic system.

Some cancers, for example, leukaemia (cancer of the blood) occur where a number of abnormal blood cells are manufactured in the bone marrow and circulate in the blood stream: not all cancers are solid cancers.

Metastases

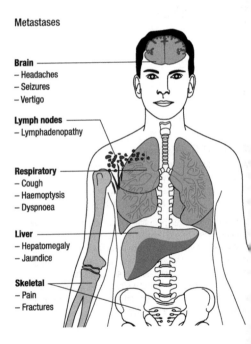

Brain
– Headaches
– Seizures
– Vertigo

Lymph nodes
– Lymphadenopathy

Respiratory
– Cough
– Haemoptysis
– Dyspnoea

Liver
– Hepatomegaly
– Jaundice

Skeletal
– Pain
– Fractures

■ HOW MALIGNANT TUMOURS GROW AND SPREAD

When cancer has metastasesed and affected other parts of the body, the disease is still referred to the organ of origination; for example, if a cancer of the cervix metastaseses to the lungs then it is still called cervical cancer, not lung cancer. Most cancers develop and spread via an organ, but blood cancer such as leukaemia does not; this affects the blood and the organs that form blood (for example the bone marrow) and then invades nearby tissues.

A developing cancer

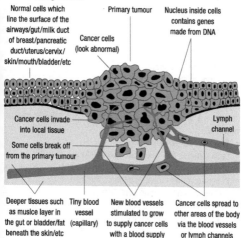

Normal cells which line the surface of the airways/gut/milk duct of breast/pancreatic duct/uterus/cervix/skin/mouth/bladder/etc

Primary tumour

Nucleus inside cells contains genes made from DNA

Cancer cells (look abnormal)

Cancer cells invade into local tissue

Lymph channel

Some cells break off from the primary tumour

Deeper tissues such as muslce layer in the gut or bladder/fat beneath the skin/etc

Tiny blood vessel (capillary)

New blood vessels stimulated to grow to supply cancer cells with a blood supply

Cancer cells spread to other areas of the body via the blood vessels or lymph channels

Source: Egton Medical Information Services

■ LOCAL GROWTH AND DAMAGE TO NEARBY TISSUES

Malignant cells multiply quickly needing a blood supply to obtain oxygen, nutrients and remove waste for new and separating cells: without a blood supply there will be no growth. The immune system has to fail to recognise or respond to the tumour. Malignant cells have a number of properties, for example:

- the ability to push through or between normal cells, dividing and multiplying
- causing damage to the local surrounding tissue as they invade it

A number of host characteristics will impact on tumour growth:

- age
- sex
- overall health status
- immune system function

Age

Cancer is a disease of older people: incidence rates increase with age.

- Few cancers are found in children.
- Leukaemia is the most common childhood cancer.
- Most common cancer in young men is testicular cancer.
- In young women most common cancers are malignant melanoma and Hodgkin Lymphoma.
- One in ten cancers are diagnosed in 25–49 year olds.
- Common cancers in females aged 25–49 years old are breast cancer, malignant melanoma and cervical cancer.

- In men aged 25–49 years the common cancers are testicular cancer, malignant melanoma and colorectal cancer.
- Those aged between 50 and 74 years are mostly affected by cancer.
- Over half of all cancers are diagnosed in 50–74 year olds.
- In men prostate cancer, lung cancer and colorectal cancers are most common.
- Most common cancers in females are breast, lung and colorectal cancer.
- Over a third of all cancers are diagnosed in the elderly population.
- Common cancers in 75 years plus in men are prostate, lung and colorectal cancers; in females these are breast, colorectal and lung cancers.

Sex

Certain cancers are more prevalent in one sex than in the other. Sex hormones influence tumour growth in:

- breast
- endometrial
- cervical
- prostate cancers

In general, it is acknowledged that men are significantly at greater risk of getting all the common cancers that occur in both sexes and dying from them more than their female counter-parts.

Overall health status

A person's overall health status can impact on tumour growth. The demand made on the body can lead to cachexia (wasting syndrome). Chronic tissue trauma requires cells to multiply and divide as healing occurs, the more rapidly cells divide the more likely there will be cellular mutation, therefore any form of chronic tissue trauma will have an impact on tumour growth.

Immune system function

Cells and organs of the immune system work together to defend the body against attack by foreign or non-self invaders. The immune system helps prevent diseases including cancer and recognises the difference between cells that are healthy and cancerous working to eradicate cancerous cells. If for any reason the immune system fails to function adequately this makes the host more susceptible to tumour growth.

■ SPREAD TO THE LYMPHATIC SYSTEM AND THE LYMPH NODES

There are some malignant cells that can enter the local lymph; the body has a network of lymph channels draining the lymphatic fluid.

The lymphatic system

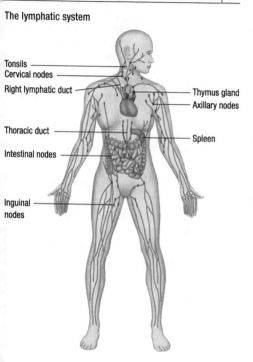

Tonsils
Cervical nodes
Right lymphatic duct
Thoracic duct
Intestinal nodes
Inguinal nodes

Thymus gland
Axillary nodes
Spleen

Source: from Colbert, B.J., Ankey, J. and Lee, K.T. *Anatomy and Physiology for Health Professionals. An Interactive Journey*, 1st. Printed and electronically reproduced by permission of Pearson Education, Inc., Upper Saddle River, New Jersey.

A malignant cell can be carried to a lymph node and become trapped, multiply and develop into a tumour. When a lymph node is in close proximity to a tumour the lymph node can enlarge, containing cancerous cells.

■ SPREAD TO OTHER PARTS OF THE BODY

Malignant cells can enter the capillary network (a network of small blood vessels), and can then be transported in the bloodstream to other parts of the body. They may multiply forming secondary tumours in one or more parts of the body; these can then grow, invade and injure adjacent tissues and spread again.

BENIGN TUMOURS	MALIGNANT TUMOURS
Non cancerous	Cancerous
May grow large and compress adjoining tissue/organs	Potential to destroy nearby tissue
Slow spreading	Fast rate of spread
Does not grow abnormally	Grows abnormally
Usually encapsulated	Non encapsulated
Differentiated	Undifferentiated
Usually non life threatening (has the potential to become malignant)	Can be life threatening

■ SECTION SUMMARY

Malignant and benign are two terms associated with cancer that can often be confused with each other; however they are different in meaning. Malignant refers to cancerous cells and can invade the tissues close to the surrounding area and spread. Benign tumours are not cancerous; they can grow in size but, do not spread.

There are many characteristics within the host that can affect tumour growth, for example, age, sex, overall health status and immune function.

Aetiology of cancer

The causes of most cancers remain unknown.
- A minority of cancers are known to be hereditary (inherited), for example, some breast cancers.
- Some people are born with a gene mutation inherited from their mother or father, increasing the risk, but they do not increase the risk for every kind of cancer; not everyone born with a gene change will develop cancer. This is referred to as hereditary cancer.
- When cancer occurs because of an inherited gene mutation risk increases: this is termed genetic susceptibility.
- Cancers not inherited are known as sporadic cancers.
- Most cancers do not have any obvious hereditary cause.
- People with an inherited gene change have a 50% chance of passing the mutation to each of their children.

Cancer is a common disease, so most families will have some members who have had cancer, but that does not mean the cancer in that family is hereditary. It is believed that most – perhaps 90% – of all cancers are sporadic. This means that even if cancer does not run in a family, a family member can still be at risk for some type of cancer in their lifetime.

Chemicals or environmental factors: carcinogens can cause normal cells to become abnormal and cancerous by damage or they initiate a mutation of a cell's genetic material (the DNA and RNA).

- Smoking is known to increase an individual's risk of lung cancer.
- Over-exposure to ultraviolet sunlight increases the risk of melanoma.
- Inhalation of asbestos dust can cause a cancer of the lining of the lungs (mesothelioma).

Some viruses are known to be carcinogens, for example, the human papilloma virus is associated with cancer of the cervix. Also linked with cancer incidence is radiation. Other factors may influence cancer incidence such as:

- diet
- exercise
- obesity

Oncogenes are genes present in the DNA of cells carrying out a number of normal functions, but they have the ability to turn a normal cell cancerous (they are a cancer causing gene).

■ CANCER-CAUSING SUBSTANCES (CARCINOGENS)

Several agents can cause cancer in the environment: these are called carcinogens.

Smoking

Smoking tobacco is closely associated with death caused by cancer; tobacco is a very powerful carcinogen. Worldwide, smoking is the single biggest cause of cancer. The most common cancer is lung cancer, but tobacco smoking can also be strongly associated with other types of cancer, for example:

Effects of smoking

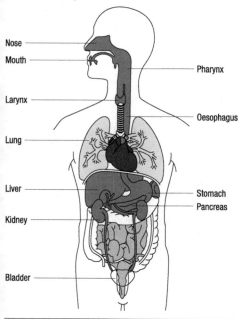

Source: Cancer Research UK

Smoking increases the risk of developing acute myeloid leukaemia (blood cancer) and cervical cancer.

Alcohol

There is a clear link between excessive alcohol consumption and the development of cancer. Alcohol consumption increases the risk of cancers of the:

- oral cavity
- pharynx
- larynx
- oesophagus
- breast
- bowel
- liver

When a person smokes and drinks heavily this will increase the risk of cancers of the upper aerodigestive tract (the upper respiratory and upper digestive tracts).

Occupational exposure

It is often very difficult to assess the role of occupational exposures in the development of cancer as cancer is caused by complex relationships of many factors. Occupational cancer can occur as a result of working environments that involve direct exposure to a carcinogen or exposure to a carcinogen produced as part of a work process.

TYPE OF EXPOSURE	INDUSTRY
Arsenic	Mining, vineyard workers, pesticide production
Asbestos	Shipbuilding, construction, mining, asbestos-producing companies
Diesel	Transportation workers/drivers, bus drivers, road maintenance, mechanics and garage workers, dockworkers
Formaldehyde	Pathologists, medical laboratory technicians, plastics, textile and plywood industry
Certain metal compounds	Iron and steel founding, house painting and paper hanging, smelting, welding
Silica	Mining, stone quarrying and granite production
Ultra violet radiation	Outdoor occupations
Wood dust	Furniture and cabinet making, construction, log and saw mill workers

Diet

It is difficult to establish the association between cancer and diet. Diet influences the risk of many cancers. Consuming high levels of fat and in particular animal fats have been linked to cancers of the:

- colon
- breast

- oesophagus
- stomach
- prostate

Eating large amounts of beef, pork and lamb may increase a person's chances of developing bowel or stomach cancer; consuming large amounts of processed meats can also increase risk. A healthy, balanced diet can boost defences against cancer.

Sun
Too much sun exposure causes cancer resulting in DNA damage and immunosuppression. Sun exposure is the main cause of skin cancer. Intense, intermittent sun exposures, such as the type experienced on holiday when sunbathing, present the greatest risk of malignant melanomas.

Hormones
The naturally occurring hormones can pose a risk to the person for developing a cancer when they are present in high levels; they encourage cells to grow and divide at a faster rate than usual.

Women with the highest levels of oestrogen and associated hormones have over twice the average risk of breast and uterine cancer, and higher risks of ovarian cancer. In men, it is still unclear if high levels of testosterone increase the risk of developing prostate cancer. Prostatic cancer cells are dependent upon testosterone. Excessive levels of insulin have been associated with cancers of the:

- colon
- uterus
- pancreas
- kidney

Staging and grading of cancer

When a person has been diagnosed with cancer they are usually told what stage the cancer is: this is a measure of how much the cancer has grown and spread. Grading refers to specific characteristics of the cancer cells: generally the earlier the stage and the lower the grade of the cancer, the better the prognosis.

■ STAGING

Staging helps the patient and the clinician decide upon the most appropriate management of the disease and how well it might respond to treatment. An international staging system is the most commonly used system for most adults presenting with solid tumours – this is known as the TNM system.

- T for tumour – how far the primary tumour has grown locally (tumour extension).
- N for nodes – if there is spread to the local lymph nodes (lymph node dissemination).
- M for metastases – if there is spread to other parts of the body (distant tumour spread).

After a cancer has been staged, a number is given for each of the three characteristics. In a man with stomach cancer, for example, the following could apply:

Tumour	• T-1 the primary tumour is still in the stomach wall • T-3 the primary tumour has grown right through the wall of stomach • T-4 the tumour is invading nearby structures, for example, the pancreas
Nodes	• N-0 there has been no spread to the lymph nodes • N-1 some local lymph nodes have been affected • N-2 there has been a more extensive spread to local lymph nodes
Metastases	• M-0 there are no metastases • M-1 there are metastases to some other area of the body, for example, the liver or brain

The TNM system:
• allows clinicians to assess a person's prognosis
• ensures that all healthcare professionals are using a standardised system
• can be seen as providing a bench mark on which to make further judgment

The table below gives a fuller explanation of the TNM system that can be applied to most cancers; this is how you may see other healthcare professionals documenting or discussing the staging of the cancer.

T (TUMOUR SIZE)

T0	No evidence of primary tumour
TI, II, III, IV	The number is allocated to the size of the primary tumour, with 'I' representing the smallest size working upwards to 'IV' the largest size
TX	Primary tumour unable to be assessed

N (regional lymph node involvement)

N0	No evidence of regional lymph node involvement
NI, II, III, IV	The number is allocated to the involvement of the regional lymph nodes, with 'I' denoting confinement to one group, working upwards to 'IV' when several groups are involved
NX	Regional lymph nodes unable to be assessed

M (distant metastases)

M0	No evidence of distant metastatic spread
MI	Evidence of metastatic spread
MX	Distant metastases cannot be assessed

Below is a diagrammatic representation of a TNM classification for a colon cancer.

Dysplasia

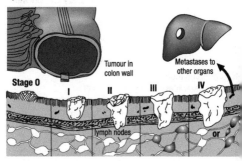

Understandably, patients may be very anxious after they have been given a diagnosis of cancer and as soon as possible after initial diagnosis they should be told about the stage of their cancer. Investigations will be carried out to determine the stage and during this time the nurse should:

- offer support to the patient and their family
- make referrals to appropriate organisations, for example, Macmillan

You are already aware that the TNM staging system is commonly used with adults with solid tumours. Other types of classifications exist and are used, for example, for malignant melanoma: a scale called the 'primary tumour thickness scale', also known as the Breslow thickness.

Haematological tumours are not solid tumours and the TNM classification is unsuitable due to the systematic nature of these malignancies. Other classification systems are used, for example:

CANCER	CLASSIFICATION SYSTEM
Hodgkin lymphoma	Ann Arbor system
Myelobastic leukaemia	French, American, British (FAB) system or the World Health Organization system
Chronic lymphoblastic leukaemia	Rai system

■ STAGING AND INVESTIGATIONS

After a diagnosis a number of tests and investigations will be needed to determine the stages. The type of investigation or test will vary subject to the cancer and may include blood tests and scans. The range of investigations falls into three key groups:

- radiology
- pathology
- endoscopy

Radiology

Using radiological investigation allows for visualisation of internal body structures. A number of X-rays (gamma rays) are used to generate an image of the body, for example, a mammogram. Sometimes a contrast medium is used, for example, if an image of the gastro intestinal tract is required the patient will be asked to swallow a contrast medium that enhances the structures of the gastro intestinal tract.

- Computerised Tomography Scan (CT Scan)
- Magnetic Resonance Imaging (MRI)
- Ultrasound
- Positron Emission Tomography (PET)

Pathology

Pathological tests include tests on body fluids, for example, blood and urine. Biochemical tests can confirm normal or abnormal levels of various chemicals, for example, alkaline phosphate. Tumour markers (usually proteins) are produced by a tumour or by the body as it makes a response to cancer. There are some tumour markers that will only be produced by one type of cancer; others can be made by many cancer types. Some markers can be found in cancerous and non-cancerous conditions.

A biopsy can be used for histological examination; this is analysed microscopically to determine if the cells are normal or cancer cells. Sometimes biopsies are able to tell where in the body a cancer has started. In some types of cancer it is virtually impossible to diagnose cancer any other way.

Endoscopy and surgery

Endoscopy may be needed to enable samples of suspected cancerous tissue to be retrieved for analysis. The figure shows a colonoscopy.

Colonoscopy

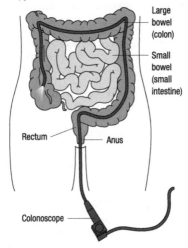

Large bowel (colon)

Small bowel (small intestine)

Rectum

Anus

Colonoscope

Endoscopies can include:
 gastroscopy
 colonoscopy
 cystoscopy
 hysteroscopy

Surgical intervention may be needed to look inside the deeper cavities or a difficult to reach part or parts of the body. There are times when a cancer cannot be accurately staged until an operation has been performed to remove the primary tumour. The tissues removed with the tumour are analysed to see how far the cancer cells have grown through the normal tissues and whether nearby lymph nodes contain cancer cells.

The nurse has an important role to play in all of the above investigations offering support to the patient before, during and after the investigation. Some of the investigations discussed require specific pre-investigation preparation, for example:

- The patient needs to be nil by mouth for a gastroscopy.
- Jewellery and metal objects need to be removed for certain scans.
- An enema or bowel preparation may be needed for some bowel investigations.

An opportunity must be given for the patient to ask any questions if they are unsure or are seeking clarification.

■ GRADING AND INVESTIGATIONS

Grading can occur after biopsy, for instance, after microscopic examination or testing in other ways, for example, through cytological testing. In the laboratory certain features of the cells can be observed and the cancer can be graded as low, intermediate or high.

- Low-grade cancers are often slow-growing and can appear similar to normal cells (are well differentiated). These cells are often less aggressive and they are less likely to spread quickly.
- Intermediate-grade is a middle grade.
- High-grade suggests that the cancer cells are fast growing, they look very abnormal (poorly differentiated),

are likely to be more aggressive and usually spread quickly.
- Breast cancers are graded 1, 2 or 3 similar to low-grade, intermediate-grade and high-grade.
- Prostate cancer is graded by Gleason score; this is similar to other grading systems, a low Gleason score means much the same as low-grade and a high Gleason score means much the same as high-grade.

The stage and the grade are used together to advise about the various treatment options and when discussing prognosis.

■ SECTION SUMMARY

It is important to grade and classify the type of cancer (if possible). This informs treatment and provides an opportunity to discuss prognosis. Patients will be understandably anxious when diagnosed with cancer and will often ask how far advanced it is. Staging and grading allows clinicians to answer this question.

The most common classificatory system for adult solid tumours is the TNM system. For non-solid tumours, i.e. haematological tumours, other systems exist.

There are several types of tests and investigations needed to classify the stage of cancer. The nurse has a role to play in helping patients understand these tests and to ensure that they are safely prepared and cared for before, during and after the procedure.

Grading of the tumour occurs when the cells are analysed: cells are observed to determine what their features are. The cancer can then be graded as low, intermediate or high grade.

Fill in the table below regarding the care of a patient undergoing the specific investigation prior to the procedure, during the procedure and after the procedure. You should consider the physical, legal and psychological aspects of care.

INVESTIGATION	PHYSICAL	LEGAL	PSYCHOLOGICAL
Chest X-ray			
Ultrasound of the abdomen			
CAT Scan			
PET Scan			
Serum liver function tests			
Biopsy of the oesophagus			
Colonoscopy			
Laparoscopy of the ovaries			
Laparotomy			

Cancer treatment

Successful treatment depends on:
- early detection of the disease
- careful staging and grading assessing the extent of the cancer
- prompt intervention
- appropriate support
- medical and technological advances

Cancer can be treated in different ways depending on the type of cancer, where it is in the body and if it has spread.

knowing more about what the treatments involve can help the nurse care competently and confidently for the person with cancer and their family.

Cancer treatment aims to:

cure

control the disease process

offer palliation of symptoms

These goals may overlap and people are often given more than one type of treatment for their cancer. Treatment for cancer may be through:

surgery

chemotherapy

radiotherapy

biotherapy

hormonal therapy

bone marrow and stem cell transplants

Treatment options will be discussed with the patient and at multidisciplinary team meetings and relate to tumour staging and grading. The goals of treatment are:

eliminating the tumour or malignant cells

preventing metastases from developing

reducing cellular growth and tumour burden

promoting independence, functional abilities and providing pain relief to those whose disease has not responded to treatment

SURGERY

Surgery is used for the diagnosis and staging of most cancers. It is also considered for reconstruction (in breast cancer) and prophylactically. As a primary treatment for cancer, the objective is to eradicate the whole tumour, a clear margin of unaffected surrounding tissue and if lymph nodes are suspicious these are also removed. On occasion surgical intervention results in injury to the body and the formation of new structures to take over the function of structures lost during surgery; for example, in the removal of the distal sigmoid colon and rectum, an alternative means of providing elimination is required, the remaining segment of healthy colon is brought out through a created opening, a stoma on to the abdominal wall resulting in a permanent colostomy.

Side effects

- Destruction of nerves.
- Loss of normal functioning; for example, surgery on the prostate gland can lead to incontinence and erectile dysfunction.
- Surgical removal of diseased regional lymph nodes may lead to long-term lymphoedema; lymphoedema of the arm can occur after surgery for breast cancer.

When the tumour is inoperable or there is widespread metastases, surgery may be palliative:

- allowing the involved organs to function for as long as possible
- to relieve pain and provide comfort
- to bypass an obstruction

Surgery can help to reduce the bulk of the tumour enhancing the ability to control the residual disease through other treatment options, such as chemotherapy and radiotherapy. Often surgery is used in combination with other treatments to effect a cure.

Radiotherapy can be used before surgery to reduce the size of the tumour prior to being removed.

Exploratory laser technology is being considered for use in different types of cancer surgery, this:

- minimises blood loss
- decreases deformity
- enhances the accuracy of tissue resection
- promotes healing

In prostate cancer there has been an increase in laser use to preserve urinary continence and sexual functioning.

The nurse has a responsibility to help prepare the person physically, psychologically and legally for the proposed surgery; the role extends to the post-operative period teaching the person what to expect. The person should be given the opportunity to ask questions and discuss concerns and fears. There may be some instances where the person may wish to discuss alternative treatment options. In this case, the person must be listened to and their decision respected. It is imperative that the person makes an informed decision.

■ CHEMOTHERAPY

Chemotherapy is the treatment of cancer using anti-cancer drugs, cytotoxic drugs.

- Chemotherapeutic drugs can prevent cancer cells dividing and reproducing.
- The drugs are transported in the blood stream and can reach cancer cells anywhere in the body.
- They can also be taken up by some healthy cells.
- Healthy cells can repair the damage caused by chemotherapy but cancer cells cannot; they eventually die.

A number of new anti-cancer drugs are becoming available; these are known as targeted treatments. Cytotoxic drugs affect the growth of cancer cells and normal cells: the newer drugs are specifically targeted against certain parts of the cancer cells.

Cytotoxic drugs are still the most widely used form of chemotherapy. Chemotherapy agents act in a number of ways. They are:

- phase-specific, working at specific points of the cell cycle

or

- non-phase-specific; working throughout the entire cell cycle

Chemotherapeutic agents are commonly used in combination to increase the potential cell kill because tumours are made up of cells replicating at different rates, therefore, a combination of drugs affecting the cell at different points in the cell cycle has a better chance of being effective. Combinations of drugs are used when a cancer shows signs of drug resistance which develops when cells mutate rapidly.

Chemotherapy drugs can cause unpleasant side effects, as they affect some of the healthy cells in the body. Damage to the healthy cells is usually temporary: most side effects will disappear once treatment is over. Healthy cells in certain parts of the body are especially sensitive to chemotherapy drugs, including:

- bone marrow
- hair follicles
- lining of the mouth
- digestive system

t is usual for chemotherapy to be given as a series of essions of treatment, with each session followed by a rest eriod: a cycle of treatment. A series of cycles make up a ourse of treatment. With each session of chemotherapy nore of the cancer cells are destroyed; the rest period allows he normal cells and tissues to recover.

There are over 50 different cytotoxic chemotherapeutic drugs available. Combination chemotherapy can be used. he kind of chemotherapy treatment given depends on a umber of things, including:

- type of cancer
- primary site
- cancer grade
- metastatic spread

Chemotherapy can also be used with other types of reatment, for example:

- surgery
- radiotherapy
- hormonal therapy
- biological therapies

r

- a combination of these

Classes of chemotherapeutic drugs

Chemotherapeutic agents can be classified either by the effects of the agent on the cell or its pharmacological properties. Usually they are grouped as:

- alkylating agents
- antimetabolites
- anti tumour antibiotics
- mitotic inhibitors

CLASSIFICATION	ACTION
Alkylating Agents	The oldest class of agents used and are either: • Mono-functional; targeting one part of DNA formation • Bi-functional; there are two opportunities in the cell cycle of working Used to treat leukaemias, lymphomas and solid cancers Affect stem cells and may lead to infertility; other side effects are nephrotoxicity and haemorrhagic cystitis
Antimetabolites	Phase specific drugs, interfering with the making of DNA causing cells to die. Side effects occur when high levels of the drug are administered; affecting rapidly dividing cells, for example, those in the gastrointestinal tract, the hair, skin and white blood cells. Examples are: folic acid analogues (methotrexate – treats breast cancer), pyrimidine analogues (5-fluorouracil) – treats colorectal and pancreatic cancers, cytosine arabinoside (ARA-C) – treats acute myeloid leukaemia, gemcitabine – used for pancreatic cancer and purine analogues (6-mercaptopurine) – used for lymphomas and leukaemias

CLASSIFICATION	ACTION
Anti tumour antibiotics	Originally derived from natural sources, generally too toxic to be used as antibacterial agents. They are not phase specific, acting in several ways: • Disrupting DNA replication and RNA transcription • Creating free radicals, generating breaks in DNA • Interfering with DNA repair • Binding to cells, killing them They also damage the cardiac muscle, limiting the amount and duration of treatment. Examples include actinomycin D, doxorubicin, bleomycin, mitomycin-C, and mithramycin.
Mitotic inhibitors	Act to prevent cell division, include the plant alkaloids and taxoids. Plant alkaloids are extracted from plant sources: • Vinca alkaloids (e.g., vincristine and vinblastine) • Etoposide Side effects associated are: • Depression of deep tendon reflexes • Pain and altered sensation • Motor weakness • Cranial nerve disruptions • Paralytic ileus

CLASSIFICATION	ACTION
	Etoposide may cause bone marrow suppression, nausea and vomiting. The most common toxic effect is hypotension when the intravenous administration is too rapid. Taxoids act by inhibiting cell division. Paclitaxel is used for the treatment of Kaposi's sarcoma and metastatic breast and ovarian cancer. Side effects include alopecia, bone marrow depression, and severe hypersensitivity reactions, e.g. hypotension, dyspnoea and urticaria.

Side effects

Side effects vary depending on the drug used and the length of treatment. Most of the drugs act on fast-growing cells, side effects impact on normally rapidly dividing cells. Tissues usually affected by cytotoxic drugs include:

- mucous membranes of the mouth, tongue, oesophagus, stomach, intestine and rectum
- hair cells, resulting in alopecia
- bone marrow depression affecting most blood cells, results in impaired ability to respond to infection, diminished ability to clot blood and severe anaemia
- organs, such as heart, lungs, bladder, kidneys
- reproductive organs, resulting in impaired reproductive ability or altered foetal development
- nerve damage causing neuropathies and loss of sensation in the soles and palms

You must be aware of the side effects so supportive treatment can be provided; this will include physical and psychological care. You must provide patients with a safe environment, for example, ensuring risks associated with infection are reduced.

RADIOTHERAPY

Many patients choose to receive radiotherapy as part of treatment. This can be given as:

- External radiotherapy – high energy x-rays are used from outside of the body, normally given as a series of short, daily treatments using equipment similar to a large x-ray machine.
- Internal radiotherapy – a radioactive material is placed internally – inside the body and is used primarily to treat cancers of the head and neck, cervix, uterus, prostate gland or skin.

Treatment is given in one of two ways:

- Brachytherapy – solid radioactive material is placed close to or inside the tumour for a limited period of time.
- Radioisotope treatment – radioactive liquid is administered either as a drink or as an intravenous injection.

Radiotherapy works by destroying cancer cells in the area treated. However, healthy normal cells may also become damaged by radiotherapy, usually repairing themselves. Radiotherapy can cure some cancers and may also reduce the risk of a cancer recurring after surgery. It may also be used to alleviate symptoms caused by cancer.

There are specific nursing interventions required after radiotherapy:

- provision of psychological and physical support
- the site to be treated is usually marked on the skin with a semi permeable marker: this should not be washed off, otherwise all the measurements for positioning of the radiotherapy beam will have to be recalculated

The nurse should also advise the patient:
- not to wash the treated area with soap or apply creams, talcum powder or other topical preparations, as this may lead to skin damage
- avoid rubbing, scratching, shaving or exposing the area to sunlight
- not to apply hot or cold packs to the area
- to wear loose cotton clothing
- to check the skin condition daily, reporting any changes

■ BIOLOGICAL THERAPIES

Biological therapies (immunotherapy) use substances occurring naturally in the body to destroy cancer cells. There are several types of treatment:
- monoclonal antibodies
- cancer growth inhibitors
- vaccines
- gene therapy

■ BONE MARROW AND STEM CELL TRANSPLANTS

Bone marrow transplantation (BMT) is an accepted treatment stimulating a non-functioning marrow or to replace marrow. BMT is given as an intravenous infusion of bone marrow cells from a donor to the person. Most commonly used in leukaemias, this therapy is being expanded to include treatment of other cancers including melanoma and testicular cancer.

HORMONES AND HORMONE ANTAGONISTS

Hormonal therapies act by changing the production or activity of specific hormones in the body, and are most commonly used to treat breast and prostate cancers. The type of hormone therapy given depends on the type of cancer being treated. There are a number of types of hormonal therapy.

Hormone antagonists work with hormone-binding tumours of the breast, prostate and endometrium, blocking the hormone's receptor site on the tumour, preventing it from receiving normal hormonal growth stimulation. These drugs do not cure, but cause regression of the tumour in approximately 40% of breast and endometrial tumours and in 80% of prostate tumours.

Side effects can impair healing and may also lead to:
- hyperglycaemia
- hypertension
- osteoporosis
- hirsutism

SECTION SUMMARY

Broadly cancer treatment may be through:
- surgery
- chemotherapy
- radiotherapy
- biotherapy
- hormonal therapy
- bone marrow and stem cell transplants

There is no single treatment for cancer: a number of options are available and decisions are based on an individual assessment. Often a combination of several types of treatment are required ensuring greatest effect, taking into account a variety of factors, including the patient's age, history and lifestyle. At all times the patient should be at the centre of the decision making process. High quality care means that the patient is cared for in a holistic manner.

Surgery may be indicated with the aim of removing the cancer. Chemotherapy may be required before or after surgery. There may be a need for radiotherapy or other forms of treatments.

All forms of treatment have side effects, some more tolerable than others. The nurse has to provide as much information as possible to the patient so he/she is able to make a truly informed decision about care management proposals.

Take some time and think about the various types of treatment listed below and think of the potential side effects. When you have done this begin to think of ways in which the nurse can help the patient address the issues identified.

TREATMENT	POTENTIAL SIDE EFFECTS	ALLEVIATING NURSING INTERVENTIONS
Chemotherapy		
Radiotherapy		
Brachytherapy		
Hormone therapy		

Cancer fast facts

BREAST CANCER

INCIDENCE	RISK
Nearly 50,000 people are diagnosed with breast cancer each year in the UK	The biggest risk factor, after gender, is increasing age – about 81% of breast cancers occur in women over the age of 50
It is the second biggest cause of death from cancer for women in the UK, after lung cancer	Two genes BRCA1 and BRCA2 give higher risk – about 7% of women have these genes
Men can get breast cancer but, it is rare with about 300 men diagnosed annually	Smoking, regular alcohol intake, the contraceptive pill, overweight and obesity increase risk
	Having more children and breastfeeding for longer than 9 months reduces risk
	Breast cancers have been linked to oestrogen
	Women currently taking HRT have a 66% increased risk of breast cancer compared to non-users
	A woman with one affected first-degree relative (mother or sister) has nearly double the risk of breast cancer of a woman with no family history of the disease; if two (or more) relatives are affected, risk increases further

MORTALITY	SURVIVAL
Breast cancer accounts for approximately 16% of female deaths from cancer in the UK and was the most common cause of death from cancer in women until 1998; since then lung cancer causes more deaths Those aged 35–54 years, breast cancer is the most common cause of all deaths from cancer	Last 30 years survival rates for breast cancer have been improving In England for women diagnosed with breast cancer in 2001–2006, five-year relative survival rates have reached 82% compared with only 52% thirty years earlier in 1971–75

SCREENING	SYMPTOMS AND TREATMENT
Breast screening is a method of detecting breast cancer at a very early stage. The first step involves mammogram The NHS breast screening programme is extending the age range of women eligible to ages 47 to 73	Breast cancer symptoms vary widely but include: • a lump that can be felt • change in the breast size or shape • altered skin texture • drawing in of the nipple Breast lumps are, however, common, particularly in younger women; most are not cancerous. About a third of women diagnosed with breast cancer have no symptoms and are detected by breast screening Diagnosis is made by biopsy Treatment is usually multimodal and includes: • surgery • adjuvant therapy • radiotherapy • chemotherapy • endocrine therapy • biological therapy

BOWEL CANCER (ALSO KNOWN AS COLORECTAL CANCER)

INCIDENCE	RISK
39,991 people in the UK were diagnosed with bowel cancer in 2008	Incidence is generally higher in populations with 'westernised' diets, these populations also tend to have a higher percentage of overweight and obese people undertaking lower levels of exercise
It is the third most common cancer after breast and lung	
More tumours diagnosed in the left hand side of the bowel, approximately 60% of tumours occur in the sigmoid colon, rectosigmoid junction and rectum	A lower risk of colon cancer occurs with higher fibre intake
	Obesity, alcohol intake and smoking are related to an increased risk of colon cancer
More men than women have colorectal cancer	
Large bowel cancer is strongly related to age, the majority of cases arising in those 60 years or older	A small number of bowel cancers are linked to a dominantly inherited predisposition
Incidence rates across the UK vary	

MORTALITY	SURVIVAL
16,259 deaths from colorectal cancer in the UK in 2008, comprising 10,164 from colon and 6,095 from rectal cancer	Five-year relative survival rates for male and female colon and rectal cancer have doubled between the early 1970s and mid 2000s
Second most common cause of death from cancer in the UK is colorectal cancer after lung cancer	Younger patients have a better prognosis than older patients
Most deaths occur in older people, approximately 80% in those aged 65 and over and about two-fifths in the over 80s	Those diagnosed at an early stage have a much better prognosis than those who present with more extensive disease
Globally, colorectal cancer killed more than 600,000 people in 2008, more than half of these deaths reported in the more developed regions	

SCREENING

Screening can detect colorectal cancers at an early stage when survival rates are highest

Many colorectal cancers develop slowly over a number of years from adenomas, or benign polyps transforming into malignant adenocarcinomas. Screening provides the opportunity to detect and treat benign polyps before malignant transformation occurs, some polyps turn out to be cancerous when detected

Population screening using the faecal occult blood test every two years can reduce colorectal mortality by between 15% and 18% in people aged 45–74

Men and women of the relevant ages should be invited to participate every two years by using FOBT kits in their own home, returning them to laboratories for analysis

SYMPTOMS AND TREATMENT

Often the presenting features of colon cancer are non-specific, and include weight loss and anaemia due to occult blood loss

Rectal and distal colon cancers, usually present with bleeding and/or altered bowel habits, symptoms that overlap with less serious and more common conditions

About 20% of patients may present with acute bowel obstruction or peritonitis due to bowel perforation

Main form of treatment is surgery. Other treatments include:

- chemotherapy
- radiotherapy
- biological therapies

■ LUNG CANCER

INCIDENCE	RISK
About 40,800 people in the UK were diagnosed with lung cancer in 2008	Most lung cancers are caused by smoking, 90% in men and 83% in women
Globally, it is the most common cancer, with 1.61 million new cases diagnosed annually	The second most important cause of lung cancer after tobacco is radon exposure; this is a naturally occurring radioactive gas. Some of the highest natural levels in the UK are in the southwest
Until the late 1990s in the UK, lung cancer was the most frequently occurring cancer, it still accounts for around 1 in 8 new cases	Industrial exposure to certain elements increases risk, for example, arsenic and polycyclic hydrocarbons
There are more cases of lung cancer diagnosed in men, but, the numbers of women being diagnosed has increased	Outdoor air pollution maybe be a small risk
Lung cancer is rarely diagnosed in those younger than 40, the incidence rises steeply after, peaking in people aged 80–84 years. 87% of cases occur in people over the age of 60	A family history of lung cancer in a first-degree relative is associated with a two-fold increased risk, regardless of smoking

MORTALITY	SURVIVAL
6% of all deaths and 22% of all deaths from cancer in the UK are attributed to lung cancer One person dies every 15 minutes in the UK of lung cancer 75% die at age 65 and over, but due to the large numbers of lung cancer deaths overall, over 4,000 people die from lung cancer before the age of 60	Of all cancers it has one of the lowest survival outcomes, because over two-thirds of patients are diagnosed at a late stage when curative treatment is not possible A significant difference to survival rates would occur if earlier diagnosis and referral to specialist teams were made
SCREENING	**SYMPTOMS AND TREATMENT**
There are no screening programmes available	A variety of symptoms are associated with lung cancer, usually relating to the primary tumour. Common symptoms include: • cough • dyspnoea • weight loss • chest pain Haemoptysis and bone pain are also relatively common symptoms. Finger clubbing and fever may be present Surgery is the key curative treatment for Non-Small Cell Lung Cancer and is usually the treatment of choice for early stage patients Other treatments will depend on the type of lung cancer but, will include: • chemotherapy • radiotherapy

■ PROSTATE CANCER

INCIDENCE	RISK
37,051 men in the UK were diagnosed with prostate cancer in 2008	Prostate cancer risk is strongly related to age
It is the most common cancer in men in the UK, accounting for approximately a quarter of all new male cancer diagnoses	A family history of prostate cancer is a known risk factor for this disease. A history of breast cancer may also affect a man's risk, specifically if the family members were diagnosed under the age of 60
Very few cases are registered in men under 50 and about 75% of cases occur in those over 65 years. The largest number of cases occur in the 75–79 age group	In the UK, black Caribbean and black African men have about two to three times the risk of being diagnosed or dying from prostate cancer than white men. Generally, Asian men have a lower risk than the national average
At post-mortem examination it is estimated that around half of all men in their fifties have histological evidence of cancer in the prostate. Men are therefore more likely to die with prostate cancer than from it	There may be a risk associated with smoking and alcohol intake

MORTALITY	SURVIVAL
0,168 men in the UK died from prostate cancer in 2008	The last 30 years survival rates for prostate cancer have been improving and are strongly related to the stage of the disease at diagnosis
	In England survival rates have risen from 31% for patients diagnosed in 1971–75 to 77% for men diagnosed in 2001–06
	For disease confined to the prostate, five-year relative survival for patients in 1999–2002 is 90% or more, however if the disease is metastatic at presentation five-year relative survival is lower at around 30%

SCREENING	SYMPTOMS AND TREATMENT
The three tests for prostate cancer all have drawbacks, the tests include: • digital rectal examination • prostate specific antigen • transrectal ultrasound biopsy	Localised prostate cancer is usually asymptomatic but some symptoms can arise from enlargement of the prostate gland Localised prostate cancer symptoms may be the same as those for benign prostatic enlargement: • frequency • dysuria • haematuria Bladder obstruction may eventually occur if left untreated. Advanced disease may present with pain from widespread skeletal metastases, particularly back pain Many treatments have serious side-effects There is no consensus on treatment, decisions are usually based on the risk of disease progression, categorised into low, intermediate and high risk and can include: • chemotherapy • radiotherapy • endocrine therapy • biological therapy • surgery • high-intensity focused ultrasound • cryotherapy

Caring for people with cancer

Caring for people with cancer is multifaceted. The nurse should:

- be knowledgeable using an evidence base
- be caring, kind and compassionate
- provide physical and psychological support for the person and if appropriate their family

Previous sections have discussed the various types of treatment that may be offered, often in combination. A diagnosis of cancer and subsequent treatment regimens can have a significant impact on a person's (and their family's) physical and psychological wellbeing. Clear precise information is needed to help people make decisions.

At different stages of the disease the person may require different types of support, for example:

- psychological support when first diagnosed
- subsequently, physical support may be needed when the person is undergoing the various invasive and non-invasive investigations and tests

Understanding the various tests, the reasons why they are being performed and the meanings attributed to the outcomes can help the nurse help the patient.

Patient centred care means that any treatment and care offered should always take into account the needs and preferences of the person being cared for. People with cancer should be given the opportunity to make informed decisions about care and treatment; this should be done in partnership with their healthcare professionals.

- Good communication between healthcare professionals and people with cancer is essential. This should be supported by evidence-based written information adapted to the person's individual needs.
- Treatment and care, along with the information people are given about it, should be culturally appropriate.
- It should also be accessible to those people who may have additional needs such as physical, sensory or learning disabilities and to those who do not speak or read English.

If the person is in agreement, families and carers should be given the opportunity to be involved in decisions about treatment and care. Families and carers will also need to be given the information and support that they need to cope with a diagnosis and treatment associated with cancer.

Each person is unique and their cancer is unique to them. Care should reflect the needs of the person and be tailored to encompass their cancer type. Below, make a list of the appropriate resources that you might make use of to care for the person with cancer.

CANCER TYPE	RESOURCE	DESCRIPTION OF RESOURCE	NOTES
Cervix			
Prostate			
Leukaemia			
Breast (male)			
Breast (female)			
Brain			

PALLIATIVE CARE AND END OF LIFE CARE

ot all cancers are curable. Those facing life-threatening
ness such as cancer will need some form of supportive
re in addition to treatment for their illness. Palliative care
an aspect of supportive care. The management of pain
d any other symptoms along with the provision of
ychological, social and spiritual support is essential.
e aims of palliative care are to:

- affirm life and view dying as a normal process
- offer relief from pain and any other distressing symptoms
- combine the psychological and spiritual aspects of patient
  care
- provide a support system helping people live as actively as
  possible until their death
- offer a support network helping the family cope during the
  patient's illness and in their own bereavement

ere are two distinct categories of health and social care
ofessionals who provide palliative care:

- those delivering the day-to-day care in homes and in
  hospitals
- those who specialise in palliative care, for example,
  clinical nurse specialists in palliative care

ose providing day-to-day care can:

- assess the care needs of each patient and their families
  incorporating physical, psychological, social, spiritual and
  information needs
- meet those needs, while being aware of the limits of their
  knowledge, skills, and competence in palliative care
- know when to seek advice from others or refer to other
  specialist palliative care services

A number of specialist palliative care services are available and are provided by expert multidisciplinary palliative care teams, who:

- carry out assessment
- provide advice and care for patients and families in all care settings
- provide specialist in-patient facilities in hospices or hospitals for those who would benefit from on-going support and care
- co-ordinate home support for patients with complex needs who would prefer to stay at home to die

Day care facilities are also available, offering a variety of opportunities for the assessment and review of patients' needs and facilitating the provision of physical, psychological and social interventions. Specialist teams providing palliative care include:

- palliative medicine consultants
- palliative care nurse specialists
- physiotherapists
- occupational therapists
- dieticians
- pharmacists
- social workers
- those able to give spiritual and psychological support

End of life care is closely associated with palliative care:

- offering support for people who are approaching death
- helping them to live as well as possible until they die
- helping them to die with dignity

This also includes support for their family or carers.

Palliative care aims to:
help make people as comfortable as possible
relieve pain and other distressing symptoms
provide psychological, social and spiritual support
care for the whole person as opposed to just one aspect of
their care

nd of life care also covers legal issues, such as creating
lasting power of attorney so that a person or people can
take decisions about the patient's care if they are no longer
ble to do so.

Palliative care teams usually co-ordinate all services.
atients have the right to choose where they want to receive
are and where they want to die. End of life care can be
rovided to patients and their families in hospitals, care
omes, hospices and in their own home. End of life care can
st for a few days only, or it may last for months or years.

SECTION SUMMARY

ot all cancers can be cured. The reaction to a cancer
agnosis is unique for each person and how people react
variable. Some people go through some recognised
tages of grief and this can include the nurse, patient and
eir family.

Symptom control is the chief objective of palliative care,
nd of life care (closely associated with palliative care)
espects the person's choices: this may include where it is
ey wish to die. End of life care can last for a few days or
r months or years.

Grief affects people in different ways: many people have experienced grief, but it is unique to each person. People often find it difficult to define or explain the feelings they are experiencing when they are grieving.

Think of a time when you have lost something, your wallet or purse, for example, how did you feel? Did you think:

- 'I don't believe this, this is not happening to me'
- 'Why me, why is this happening to me?'
- 'If only I could find it, I promise I will be a better a person'
- 'Well it's gone'
- 'What will be will be'

Similar feelings to those above are well documented when people have had a close relative or a loved one die, they are the stages of grieving. Sometimes those diagnosed with cancer also go through the grieving process:

- 'I don't believe you – you have the diagnosis wrong' (denial)
- 'Why me, why not some nasty person, why me I am a good person, there are worse people than me in the world' (anger)
- 'If I am cured, if God cures me I promise I will devote my life to doing good for others' (bargaining)
- 'Do what you have to do I don't care anymore – I have no interest' (depression)
- 'There is nothing I can do about this so I will live what I have left of my life to the full' (acceptance)

Not all people go through all stages nor do they go through the stages in the order presented.

erminology

low is a list of words used in association with cancer along
th their meaning.

ORD	MEANING
denocarcinoma	A cancer of glandular tissue
djuvant therapy	Treatment given supplementary to the main treatment
etiology	Study of the causes of diseases
poptosis	Cell death
typical yperplasia	Benign but abnormal cells
enign	Not cancerous
iological erapy	Treatments using naturally occurring substances within the body
iopsy	Examination of tissue removed from the patient
rachytherapy	Internal radiotherapy
arcinogen	A substance that can cause cancer
arcinoma	A malignant tumour derived from epithelial tissue
arcinoma in tu	An early cancer that has not invaded (grown into) surrounding tissues
ell cycle	The highly regulated sequence of events that a cell goes though when it grows

WORD	MEANING
Chemotherapy	The treatment of disease, usually cancer, using drugs (chemical substances)
Combination chemotherapy	Treatment with more than one anticancer drug at a time
Cytology	The study of cells
Diagnostic marker	Something in the body or body fluid that can be tested for and which points to the presence of a particular type of cancer
Dyskaryosis	Microscopic abnormal appearance of a cell's nucleus. This can be classed as mild, moderate or severe. These are all phases of pre-cancerous cells that may develop into cancer if left untreated
Fine needle aspiration	A biopsy in which a very thin needle is put into a breast lump, and a sample of fluid and cells are aspirated
Histology	Microscopic study of cells or tissues
Hyperplasia	Increased growth of cells but the cells are normal
Lesions	An area of precancerous growth
Malignant	A tumour that has spread to and grows in other parts of the body

WORD	MEANING
Metastases	Cancer cells breaking away from the primary tumour spreading to other distant sites around the body forming secondary tumours
Oncogene	A mutated gene that encourages a cancer to grow. In their unmutated form, most oncogenes are involved with the regulation of cell growth and the cell cycle
Palliation	Treatment given to relieve symptoms rather than to treat the cancer
Pathology	Science of the cause and effect of diseases
Prognosis	Estimate or prediction of the outcome of a disease
Radiotherapy	Treatment for cancer that uses high-energy radiation such as x-rays to kill cancer cells
Stage	The size of a cancer and how far it has spread
Tumour	An abnormal growth of tissue can be benign or malignant
Undifferentiated	Very immature cells with no specialised role, for example, stem cells

Resources

---

http://www.cancerresearchuk.org
Cancer Research UK: Information for professionals and a useful resource for up to date statistics and current research news. The site will help to keep you up to date with all that is developing in the field of cancer.

http://wales.gov.uk/topics/health/?lang=en
Health of Wales Information Service: This Welsh government website provides a host of information concerning health related matters. The site is easy to navigate and offers links to other UK wide resources.

http://www.macmillan.org.uk
Macmillan Cancer: The support website provides useful explanations about all cancers, how they develop, the treatments used and is helpful for anyone interested in learning more about cancer. There is an education programme which is free, however you must register to access it.

http://www.mariecurie.org.uk/
Marie Curie Cancer Care is a UK charity dedicated to the care of people with terminal cancer and other illnesses. There are over 2,000 Marie Curie Nurses who work in the homes of terminally ill patients across the UK, providing practical care and support. This website has a nurses and hospices section.

http://www.ncpc.org.uk
National Council for Palliative Care: There are publications and education packages for professionals, although there

a small charge for some of the services on the website.
ere are also details of its latest campaigns. The National
ouncil for Palliative Care is instrumental in lobbying the
overnment on behalf of vulnerable people.

tp://www.endoflifecareforadults.nhs.uk

ational End of Life Care Programme website provides online
ducation about end of life care that has been developed by
xpert palliative care clinicians. The units take between 30
nd 45 minutes to complete and certificates are available on
uccessful completion.

tp://guidance.nice.org.uk

ational Institute for Health and Clinical Excellence (NICE)
ebsite provides information on NICE guidance on improving
utcomes in cancer care for England. There are technical
ocuments as well as documents and leaflets that patients
ay find useful.

tp://www.nhs.uk/Pages/HomePage.aspx

HS Choices: On this website you will find lots of really
seful information concerning specific cancers and their
eatments. It is the UK's largest health website, providing
formation that will help people make choices about their
alth.

tp://www.dhsspsni.gov.uk/nicancernetwork-may04.pdf

e Northern Ireland Cancer Network (NICaN) is working
wards the continuous improvement in the quality of cancer
re and cancer survival for the people of Northern Ireland.
aims to promote equitable provision of high quality, patient
cused and clinically effective cancer services. There are a
mber of links available on this website.

http://www.patient.co.uk

Patient.co.uk website produces useful information to people interested in health topics; it has direct links to charitable organisations like Help the Hospices which also produces educational material for healthcare professionals.

http://sign.ac.uk/

The Scottish Intercollegiate Guidelines Network (SIGN) develops evidence based clinical practice guidelines for the National Health Service (NHS) in Scotland and amongst these are guidelines related to cancer care. SIGN guidelines are derived from a systematic review of the scientific literature with the aim of improving patient-important outcomes.